PROBIOTICS *and* DIGESTIVE HEALTH

A GASTROENTEROLOGIST'S PERSPECTIVE

Eamonn M. Quigley, MD

HEALTH
P✦INT
PRESS

The information and advice contained in this book is based upon the research and personal and professional experiences of the authors. It is not intended as a substitute for consulting with a health care professional. The publisher and authors are not responsible for any adverse effects or consequences resulting from the use of any of the suggestions, preparations, or procedures discussed in this book. All matters pertaining to your physical health should be supervised by a health care professional.

Cover design: Jeannie Tudor
Editor: Lisa Kaspin
Typesetting and book design: Gary Rosenberg

Special thanks to Jeffrey Roberts of the Irritable Bowel Syndrome Self Help and Support Group for his valuable contribution to "The Probiotic Forum."

Health Point Press
4335 Van Nuys Blvd.
Sherman Oaks, CA 91403
818-788-2040

ISBN: 0-9774356-6-0

Printed in the United States of America.

10   9   8   7   6   5   4   3   2   1

Contents

Introduction

Your overall health depends on the healthy functioning of your digestive system; not only does it pull nutrients from food to nourish the body, but it participates in protecting it against disease. The bacteria that populate the digestive tract play a major role in both of these functions. This booklet describes the beneficial bacteria and how they aid in the nourishment and defense not only of the digestive tract but of the whole body. Imbalances in the types of gut flora—friendly versus harmful—can lead to digestive upsets, which, if left unchecked, can lead to far more serious health problems. One such disease is irritable bowel syndrome.

Irritable bowel syndrome, or IBS, is the most common chronic medical condition in the Western world. Approximately 40 percent of those with IBS have symptoms severe or frequent enough to disrupt their daily lives. These symptoms include abdominal pain, diarrhea, constipation, bloating, gas, and urgency of elimination. Effective pharmaceutical options for treating IBS remain limited, because the cause is unclear and therefore most medications target the symptoms instead. However, while the cause of IBS has not been clearly identified, new clinical evidence suggests that an alteration of the normal bacterial flora may be to blame, making probiotics one of the most promising strategies to recently emerge. Probiotics are live microorganisms that confer a health benefit on the host when administered in adequate amounts. Probiotics can restore and maintain a healthy balance of the flora in the gut, as well as promote the integrity of the lining of the gastrointestinal (GI) tract. In addition, the microbe strains used in probiotics may strengthen your natural defenses, helping to protect your body against the effects of pathogenic bacteria while also stimulating your body's immune system. These beneficial microorganisms also produce many of the vitamins your body needs to stay healthy.

In this booklet, you will learn how probiotics work and why they are so critical for regulating overall digestive health. In addition, you will learn of differences between probiotic strains, and the promise of some newly discovered probiotic strains—especially *Bifidobacterium infantis* 35624 (Bifantis®)—for relieving GI problems, including IBS. We will discuss what to look for in probiotic products. Finally, you will find answers to some of your most frequently asked questions concerning probiotics and digestive health.

CHAPTER 1

Gut Bacteria and Your Digestive Health

The gastrointestinal (GI) tract is generally described as a continuous tube beginning with the mouth and ending with the anus. The primary function of the GI tract is to physically and chemically break down the food that is consumed, and extract the nutrients your body needs from this food. Of equal importance, the GI tract is also partly responsible for preventing harmful substances from being absorbed into the body. This chapter describes how the gut flora plays major roles in these processes—both in nutrition and in defense against disease.

The Gut Flora "Fingerprint"

The GI tract is home to a complex ecosystem, containing 300 to 500 different species of bacteria, or flora; these bacterial cells make up more than 95 percent of the total cells in the human body. Every human being has a unique flora "fingerprint" with regard to the types and quantities of bacteria in their GI tract. This flora "fingerprint" is set during early childhood. The human fetus lives in a sterile environment, but within a few days of birth a relatively stable microflora is established in the GI tract. The first types of bacteria that colonize the GI tract are dependent on how the infant is first fed. In breast-fed infants, bacteria known as bifidobacteria comprise more than 90 percent of the gut bacteria. Because human breast milk contains substances that promote the growth of bifidobacteria in newborns, breastfeeding is beneficial and appropriate, especially since bifidobacteria play an important role in preventing colonization of the infant's GI tract by harmful bacterial species and in providing early immune benefits.

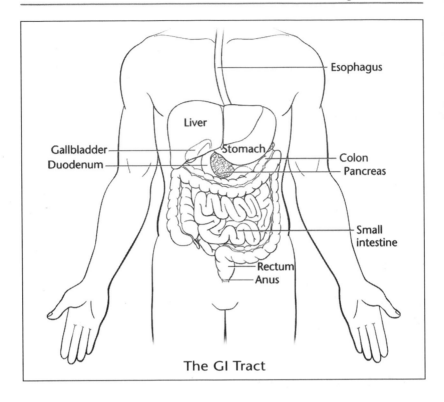

The GI Tract

Once established, the flora fingerprint changes very little throughout each person's life. In healthy people, most gut bacteria reside in
the large intestine or colon because gastric acids and intestinal movements limit the numbers of bacteria in the stomach and small intestine. Because the concentration of oxygen in the colon is very low, the
gut flora have adapted to be able to survive without oxygen or with
very little oxygen; such bacteria are, therefore, referred to as anaer-
obes. Also, the composition and location of the flora varies along the
length of the GI tract, with the greatest diversity being in the colon.
There are numerous ways bacteria can be found in this space: bacteria can be bound to food throughout the digestive process, they can
be floating free within the inner space of this tube (called the lumen),
they can be entrenched in the mucous layer that coats and protects
the intestinal tissue, and finally certain bacteria are able to attach to
the cells on the surface of the intestinal lining (called the epithelium).

Function of Gut Flora

The normal gut flora supports a variety of intestinal functions. First, the constituents of the flora play a key role in nutrition. In addition to synthesizing vitamins such as thiamine (B_1), folic acid (B_9), pyridoxine (B_6), and vitamin K, they also produce digestive enzymes and help with the absorption of nutrients (such as calcium, magnesium, and iron).

A normal gut flora also helps maintain the integrity of the colon lining, sometimes called the epithelial barrier or the mucosal barrier. The surface of the GI tract represents the human body's largest contact area with the external environment. The total surface area of the GI tract is calculated to be 150 to 200 meters square compared to the approximately 2 meters square surface of the skin. This surface is highly specialized for its primary functions—digesting food and absorbing nutrients—while also serving as a complex site of interaction with foreign substances and microorganisms introduced from the external environment during the normal course of daily life. Beneficial gut bacteria help keep this lining healthy by converting unabsorbed dietary sugars into short-chain fatty acids (SCFA), providing the major source of energy for these epithelial cells. So long as the gut epithelial barrier remains intact, harmful organisms and toxins in the lower GI tract will be unable to pass into the bloodstream or exert otherwise undesirable effects.

A third function of the normal gut flora is support and stimulation of the immune system. Beneficial bacteria in the gut work to prevent harmful bacteria from colonizing the GI tract by competing directly for space and crowding out the pathogens. The gut flora produces a variety of substances that can inhibit, or even kill, potentially harmful bacteria. In addition, they stimulate the immune system, and work in concert with the body so that the host learns to recognize these beneficial bacteria as "friendly" bacteria, therefore allowing the flora and the host to live together in a peaceful and mutually beneficial co-existence. The flora also stimulates the secretion of immunoglobulin A, a very important molecule in preventing infection. Through these immunological effects, the gut flora is also believed to assist in preventing allergies.

How Imbalances in Gut Flora Can Lead to Disease

Scientists are just beginning to understand the consequences of disruption of the delicate balance of the digestive microflora. Though the "flora fingerprint" is relatively stable throughout most peoples' lives, it can be temporarily disrupted by diet, climate changes, stress, illness, aging, and the use of certain medications, primarily antibiotics. Broadspectrum antibiotics, especially when used over the long term, can knock out many of the normal flora, setting the stage for the proliferation of competing, possibly disease-causing, organisms that are often resistant to these agents. Pathogenic and opportunistically pathogenic organisms are always present to some extent in the GI tract. The beneficial bacteria outnumber these potentially harmful bacteria and as such, the quantity of toxins produced by these bacteria has little effect on the host in a normal, healthy state. When the beneficial and harmful bacteria levels become imbalanced, this is referred to as dysbiosis, which can lead to episodes of digestive upsets in the short term and set the stage for the development of disease. The classic example of this is antibiotic-associated diarrhea and its deadliest manifestation, *Clostridium difficile* colitis. In this state *C. difficile* (a pathogenic organism that may be present in the normal GI tract at insufficient numbers to cause problems) produces two chemical toxins that directly damage the epithelium of the colon. It is, therefore, one of the most feared hospital-acquired infections and has resulted in devastating outbreaks in hospitals and nursing homes. The fact that diarrhea and *C. difficile* colitis can be prevented by the administration of a probiotic with an antibiotic (the clinical data are described in Chapter 4) provides further evidence for the protective role of the flora in this context.

In other examples of bacterial imbalance, bacteria may simply be in the wrong place. If the normal contractions of the bowel (called peristalsis or motility) are impaired and/or acid secretion from the stomach is reduced, colon bacteria may migrate upward and overpopulate the small intestine. This can interfere with proper digestion of food and absorption of nutrients. There is evidence suggesting that such overgrowth can result in symptoms that are similar to irritable bowel syndrome (IBS), especially bloating. This role of gut bacteria in IBS will be further described in Chapter 2, along with approaches to treating this common disease.

Irritable Bowel Syndrome: Finding Causes and Treatments

rritable bowel syndrome, or IBS, is the most common chronic medical condition in the Western world. Surveys of Western populations show that today between 15 and 20 percent of all adolescents and adults suffer from IBS.[1] In the United States IBS is second only to the common cold as the leading cause of absenteeism in the workplace.[2] Approximately 40 percent of those with IBS have symptoms severe or frequent enough to disrupt their daily lives (for example, work and social activities).[3] These symptoms include abdominal pain, diarrhea, constipation, bloating, gas (flatulence), and urgency of elimination.

Though there has been significant progress in our understanding of IBS and even towards better ways of making the diagnosis, IBS is all too often a "diagnosis of exclusion," meaning that it is diagnosed not by what it is, but rather by what it is not. In other words, if no underlying physiological cause for bowel symptoms can be clearly identified, an individual will receive a diagnosis of IBS. In order to diagnose a patient with IBS, a physician must first rule out alternative causes of changes in bowel health such as Crohn's disease, celiac disease, or pancreatic cancer.

In the past, few distinctions were made among IBS patients in terms of symptoms. Patients with constipation or diarrhea could receive a diagnosis of IBS. More recently, IBS has been subcategorized into diarrhea-predominant and constipation-predominant types. A group of GI specialists met in Rome, Italy, and developed the "Rome Diagnostic Criteria" for diagnosing IBS according to symptoms.[4] The current standard is the third version of these criteria that continue to evolve as we learn more.

Because there is no known cause of IBS, historically treatments for IBS have aimed to manage the symptoms. Many patients report inadequate relief after taking common IBS medications, which include antispasmodics, anti-diarrhea agents, and laxatives. In addition, taking a product to relieve one symptom may lead to or even exacerbate other symptoms.

ROME III DIAGNOSTIC CRITERIA

Recurrent abdominal pain or discomfort at least 3 days/month in the last 3 months associated with two or more of the following:

1. Improvement with defecation

2. Onset associated with a change in frequency of stool

3. Onset associated with a change in form (appearance) of stool

Causes of and Therapies for IBS

Since IBS has been defined as a cluster of symptoms with no known anatomical or physiological cause, many physicians since the 1970s came to link IBS with the psychological conditions of their patients. While these doctors often recommended medications to manage the symptoms, their primary approach was to advise their IBS patients to lower their stress levels or to seek psychological counseling. With the most recent Rome findings, the importance of the brain-gut interaction is recognized, promoting a more holistic approach tailored to the needs of each patient.

The use of antidepressants to treat IBS began as a result of studies conducted in the 1990s that examined the connections between the brain and the gut. These studies indicated that IBS patients have a lower threshold for gut pain than healthy people. In certain studies, some antidepressants (especially tricyclics, such as amitriptyline) had numbing effects on the spine pain fibers and could slow down bowel movements, which provided relief from pain. Pain relief has been observed with these agents at doses lower than those used to treat depression. However, not all patients benefit from antidepressants, and their effects in an individual patient are difficult to predict. Furthermore, these drugs can cause side effects such as drowsiness and altered brain function. While these medications may prove helpful in some patients, they are clearly not the solution to IBS for the majority of sufferers, and importantly, have not been approved by the FDA for this indication.

Another theory of IBS involves the levels of serotonin in the gut. Serotonin, which is secreted by the gut walls, controls the rate of peristalsis, or forward movement in the gut. Too much serotonin causes the gut to move too fast, resulting in diarrhea, while too little serotonin causes the gut to move too slowly, resulting in constipation. To address such findings, pharmaceutical companies developed drugs that affect serotonin receptors in the gut. But these drugs have also been shown to cause serious adverse effects. For example, the serotonin blocker alosetron, used to treat diarrhea, was removed from the market due to an increased risk of ischemic colitis, or insufficient blood flow to the colon. Tegaserod, used to treat constipation (including IBS patients with constipation), was taken off the market due to increased risk of heart attack, stroke, and worsening chest pain that could develop into heart attack.[5]

In 1994, another theory for IBS was proposed that involved bacteria: "post-infectious IBS." This theory stemmed from observations that in up to 20 percent of IBS patients, their symptoms were preceded by an acute episode of food poisoning or traveler's diarrhea. Researchers also found that some patients with infections involving microbes such as the bacteria *Campylobacter, Salmonella,* and *Shigella,* as well as parasites such as amoeba and giardia, later developed IBS. A 2002 study confirmed that 57 percent of people who developed IBS after a bout of food poisoning still met the Rome criteria for IBS six years later.[6] Research also shows that the longer and more severe the original event of food poisoning or infection, the more likely a person is to develop IBS.

It has been suggested that symptoms like those in IBS may be related in some patients to the presence of excessive numbers of bacteria in the small intestine and especially those bacteria which are normally confined to the colon, called "small intestinal bacterial overgrowth." It has been proposed that symptoms can be improved, in some patients, by a course of antibiotics. Research into this area needs to be confirmed and as such, this approach is controversial—and importantly, no antibiotics have been approved for this indication. Additionally, antibiotic-based regimens are not without their shortcomings. Overuse of antibiotics can eliminate the beneficial bacteria along with the harmful bacteria. Furthermore, resistant strains of bacteria may develop that can significantly reduce the effectiveness of subsequent antibiotic therapy. Even so, these findings provide further indication that alterations in the bacterial population of the gut play a role in the development of symptoms like those experienced in IBS.

There is a promising alternative to these more conventional medications for treating IBS and other GI problems. This alternative involves probiotics, and is based on the important role of these beneficial bacteria in promoting overall digestive health that was described in Chapter 1.

Probiotics have been defined by the World Health Organization as "live microorganisms that when administered in adequate amounts confer health benefits on the host." Probiotics are supplied in natural supplements in the form of powders, capsules or tablets. Probiotics may also be available in foods. The microbe strains found in probiotic products can protect the body against pathogens, stimulate the immune system, produce essential vitamins, and maintain the integrity of the gut lining—the epithelial barrier.

What does this mean for people with IBS? Studies have shown that shifts in the bacterial population are present in patients with IBS when compared with healthy people, with the levels of bifidobacteria in particular being lower in these individuals. To correct this imbalance, scientists are focusing on carefully formulated probiotic supplements that, when taken regularly, can significantly improve digestive health. Clinical evidence now shows that a purified strain of bifidobacteria, *Bifidobacterium infantis* 35624 , may reduce many of the symptoms associated with IBS, including pain, both diarrhea and constipation, and bloating, without undesirable side effects.[7,8]

In the next chapter, we will discuss how specific strains of probiotics can restore the proper microbial environment in the GI tract.

CHAPTER 3

Probiotics
and Digestive Health

The use of probiotics can be traced back as early as 77 A.D., when the Roman historian Plinio advocated the use of fermented milk for the treatment of GI infections.[9] Much later, in 1908, probiotics were described by the Russian scientist and Nobel laureate Eli Metchnikoff; he observed that people living in a certain part of Bulgaria who consumed fermented milk products on a regular basis had exceptional longevity. Metchnikoff concluded that the consumption of fermented milk helped to "seed" the intestine with friendly bacteria, thereby suppressing the growth of harmful bacteria. He was the first to suggest that it would be possible to modify the gut flora by replacing harmful microbes with useful microbes. These useful microbes have since become known as probiotics, which means "for life."

Probiotics are beneficial live bacteria that can aid digestion, produce essential vitamins and hormones, help strengthen the body's natural defenses, and support a more appropriate balance of healthy bacteria in the GI tract. Originally probiotics were thought to serve these functions primarily by displacing pathogenic organisms in the gut. Recent research has revealed several other effects of probiotics that could have important benefits in a variety of disorders and diseases, including IBS. It has also become clear that different strains of probiotics are unique in their effects on the body. Some provide a natural defense against pathogens, while others can help reduce inflammation that may be

It has also become clear that different strains of probiotics are unique in their effects on the body.

triggered by a flora imbalance. Still others have been shown to improve the integrity of the gut lining, preventing harmful microorganisms from passing through it into the bloodstream.

The definition of probiotics provided by the Food and Agriculture Organization of the United Nations and endorsed by many probiotic organizations such as the International Scientific Association for Probiotics and Prebiotics deserves special attention: *"probiotics are live microorganisms, which when administered in adequate amounts confer a health benefit on the host."*[10] In other words, to be really considered as a true probiotic, the organism must be live and must have been demonstrated to be beneficial in man. Nowadays the gold standard for the demonstration of clinical efficacy in humans is the randomized, double-blind, placebo-controlled clinical trial.

Probiotic bacteria are commonly found in soured (fermented) milk products such as yogurt, kefir, and cottage cheese. While some yogurt products contain enough probiotic cultures to provide health benefits, in the United States yogurt is currently not required to contain any viable probiotic cultures. Because no such requirement exists, results from tests of yogurt products sold in the United States show a wide range in the levels of viable bacteria. In addition, fermented milk products need cold storage and have a shorter shelf life than do probiotic supplements. Further, many people with digestive disorders, such as intolerance to lactose, who might benefit from probiotics cannot consume sufficiently large quantities of dairy products or do not want the calories associated with consumption of these products in the amounts that have been associated with health benefits.

Consequently, a variety of supplements have been developed to isolate and concentrate the health benefits of probiotic organisms into a form that is easier to take. Over the years, many products labeled as "probiotics" have appeared on health food store and supermarket shelves throughout the world. However, very few of these products provide any meaningful health benefits, due to a variety of reasons:

1. The benefits of a given product are often touted on the basis of evi-

dence involving different organisms than the ones contained in the product. Detailed studies have demonstrated that benefits of probiotics are very strain specific.

2. Even when the product does contain the same strain of organism that was shown to provide health benefits, it may not contain live organisms or may not have been adequately tested to ensure that the organisms will survive in storage conditions (e.g. room temperature) or for an adequate length of time. Many of these products' labels do not indicate how many organisms are in the product, or they state only "at the time of manufacture."

3. The products may not have been adequately tested in a human population.

4. The products may not contain the organism or the dose shown on the label. Analysis of some store products showed that organisms claimed on the label to be alive were actually dead. Of even more concern, a number of these products also contained organisms not mentioned on the label, in some cases including potentially pathogenic bacteria.

5. The products may not contain organisms that are resistant to bile and gastric acids, and thus would not survive passage through the GI tract to the colon.

6. The products may not contain organisms that can stick to the mucosa of the intestinal walls, which is necessary for many probiotics' health benefits.

7. The products may contain a probiotic formulation as a mixture or "cocktail": a combination of two or more bacterial strains that will theoretically maximize the individual effects of these organisms. However, the vast majority of these mixtures have not been tested in this blended form. Many probiotics in combination can block, rather than enhance, each other's benefits in certain situations, potentially minimizing the overall impact of the product.

Unfortunately, few probiotic preparations have been characterized and formulated rigorously enough to allow the manufacturer to answer these critical questions. Of further concern, critical examinations of commercially available probiotics have raised serious issues about the quality of some of these products, with independent tests finding they may contain bacteria that are not the same as those on the label. Finally, even fewer products meet the standard for complete characterization of their microbiological properties or immunological or physiological effects—and only a handful have been subjected to clinical trial in humans.

The lactic acid bacteria lactobacilli and bifidobacteria are the most abundant microorganisms in probiotic-containing foods and supplements. However, not all strains of these probiotics have similar effects. In fact, experts widely recognize that it is never appropriate to use benefits shown for one strain of bacteria to support benefits from other—even closely related—strains. Therefore, each strain must be independently tested: the gold standard to show health benefits is a double-blind, placebo-controlled clinical trial that is published in a peer-reviewed medical journal. Also, because the digestive environment is relatively stable, probiotic supplementation in the short term is unlikely to permanently change the composition of the flora. This means that continued use of probiotic supplements is necessary to sustain their health benefits.

> *. . . it is never appropriate to use benefits shown for one strain of bacteria to support benefits from other—even closely related—strains.*

When properly tested, manufactured, and consumed on a regular basis, probiotic supplements can restore and maintain gut health. They are a means of correcting an imbalance in the GI tract. Moreover, reviews of the safety of lactobacilli and bifidobacteria have concluded that they pose no health risks for consumers. Other strains, however, are of more concern as certain strains of these families of bacteria (for example, *Streptococcus*, *Enterococcus* and *Escherichia*) are known to be pathogenic.

In the next chapter, we'll consider how select probiotics have proved clinically helpful as a treatment for IBS as well as for other GI conditions.

CHAPTER 4

Probiotics for Irritable Bowel Syndrome and Other Health Conditions

Given that there are so few conventional medical treatments that effectively help to manage IBS, people who suffer from IBS often turn to alternative remedies and practices. The most common of these are dietary changes, ranging from exclusion diets to diets supplemented with a variety of dietary supplements. The concept of probiotic use in IBS has begun to find its way into the realm of conventional medicine. Properly assessing the potential role of these agents for IBS is therefore timely and important.

In this chapter we will review studies of probiotics for IBS and evaluate the potential for probiotic treatment to address possible underlying causes of IBS, including changes in the gut flora, immune activation, gut motility, and disruptions of the brain-gut axis. We will also briefly review the data on probiotics and their potential benefits for other digestive diseases.

Clinical Studies in Irritable Bowel Syndrome

A small number of clinical trials have evaluated the response of IBS symptoms to probiotic preparations and have provided limited evidence of symptom improvement. The overall impact of probiotics in IBS remains unclear, as most of the studies before 2005 were very small and therefore were not sufficiently designed. These studies had other issues besides their small size: several did not verify whether the bacteria in the products were even alive. Many different organisms and strains were tested and the amounts of bacteria in the supplement used ranged from very small amounts—100,000 bacterial colony forming units (CFUs) (10^5)—to very large amounts—more than 100 billion CFUs (10^{11}); and some employed probiotic "cocktails" that were never studied individually as single strains, making it difficult to tell which strains had the most benefit.

Nevertheless, some positive results have been noted, and recent studies have been larger and more appropriately designed. While some probiotic strains have been associated with positive results for select symptoms—*L. plantarum* 299V for abdominal pain relief, and several strains (*Lactobacillus GG, L. plantarum* (DSM 9843) and the mixture VSL#3) for reduction in bloating—no probiotic has provided effective global relief of IBS symptoms until the studies with the probiotic strain *Bifidobacterium infantis* 35624 (Bifantis). These studies are discussed in detail in Chapter 5.

Changes in the Gut Flora in IBS

Various studies have shown changes in the gut flora in IBS patients; most consistently, a decrease in the population of bifidobacteria. Such changes could lead to the growth and spread of bacterial species that produce more gas and different short chain fatty acids (SCFA). As mentioned in Chapter One, the SCFA produced by the beneficial bacteria provide energy to some of the intestinal cells and are important for their health. However, changes in the concentration of these substances can result in changes to the motility of the gut. Additionally, some bacteria change the concentration and metabolism of bile acids, which then can affect water and electrolyte transport in the colon. Because these changes can occur from an imbalance in the floral composition, they could be reversed by adding back bifidobacteria through the use of probiotics.

Probiotics can minimize the effects of pathogens in a number of ways:

- Production of bacteriocins, proteins that kill or inhibit the growth of harmful bacteria

- Production of proteases, enzymes which break down proteins (in this case, bacterial toxins)

- Competitive exclusion, based on the preferential ability of probiotics to stick to cells in the colon lining, thus keeping away harmful bacteria

As we discussed in Chapter 2, there is now a considerable body of evidence that supports the theory of post-infectious IBS. An effective probiotic could therefore help to prevent IBS that follows an attack of bacterial gastroenteritis, especially among high-risk individuals. In addition, the demonstrated anti-viral properties of some probiotic organisms, together with evidence of effectiveness of certain probiotics as a treatment for rotavirus diarrhea, suggest that probiotics could play a broader role in treating bowel dysfunctions triggered by harmful bacteria, viruses, and other infectious agents.

Immune Activation

It has been estimated that between 60 and 80 percent of the immune system components can be found in the gut, making it natural for scientists to look for a link between the most common digestive disorder, IBS, and the immune system. Recently, very exciting evidence shows this link may in fact be there.

The immune cells in the body fight infection. One way these cells react to the presence of potential pathogens is through inflammation. While inflammation is a small part of a very complex immune response, measuring the messengers the immune system uses to control inflammation (cytokines) can provide insights to help understand the linkage between immune activation and the development of IBS. The results of several small studies have provided new areas for research into the basis for this linkage:

- Studies of patients that have developed IBS following an infection have shown persistent, though subtle, inflammation in the lining of the colon walls, triggered by the continued presence of immune cytokines long after the infection is resolved. This inflammation is so subtle that it does not show up during routine biopsies (for example, those done during colonoscopy).

• Evaluations of IBS patients have found these messengers of inflammation (cytokines) in colon tissue samples as well as blood and serum samples.

• Interestingly, even though the common belief is that IBS with diarrhea is more likely to be associated with past infection, IBS with constipation has also been associated with sustained low-level inflammation of the colonic mucosa.

These findings are important as they help explain recent observations that certain types of probiotic bacteria can influence the secretion of these chemical messengers, thereby providing a rationale for the use of select strains of bifidobacteria in managing IBS.

A study published in *Gastroenterology* in 2005 provided the first definitive link between IBS and altered immune messengers (cytokines), and, importantly, was also the first study to show the benefit of certain probiotics.[7] This study demonstrated that people suffering from IBS had a different balance of cytokines than did healthy individuals, with the ratio of these messengers shifted towards a state of inflammation. The ratio of these messengers, cytokine IL-10 (an anti-inflammatory cytokine) and cytokine IL-12 (a pro-inflammatory cytokine) was normalized following eight weeks of supplementation with the probiotic strain *Bifidobacterum infantis* 35624. At the same time, their IBS symptoms (pain, bloating and bowel movement difficulty) also improved. In this same study, a strain of lactobacillus did not impact the cytokine ratio or provide symptom relief. This study shows that certain strains of probiotics may actually impact not just the symptoms of the IBS, but also a potential cause of the problem— and, importantly, shows that the benefits of probiotic bacteria are strain specific.

Additional studies paint a bit more of the picture. The probiotic cocktail (or blend of strains) called VSL#3 (which contains *Streptococcus thermophilus*, several species of lactobacillus, and bifidobacteria) can not only prevent an inflammatory GI condition known as pouchitis but can help reduce relapse rates among patients successfully treated with antibiotics for this condition. Pouchitis is a type of colitis that occurs in patients with inflammatory bowel disease (IBD) who have undergone a specific surgical procedure where the colon is removed and a "pouch" is formed from the lower part of the small intestine.

In recent efforts to understand how this blend of probiotics works, VSL#3 was shown to promote secretion of cytokine IL-10 and to suppress secretion of cytokine IL-12 (similar to what was shown in the study we discussed above). What was truly fascinating is that upon further analysis, in which the investigators evaluated each of the strains in the mixture, they found that the bifidobacteria in the cocktail were responsible for most of these effects—and that some of the other strains had just the opposite effect! Once again, this shows that all probiotic strains are not alike. Therefore strains in mixtures need to be evaluated on an individual basis as well as in the final blend.

Neuromuscular Dysfunction In The Gut

For decades, abnormal gut motility (contractions that are either too fast or too slow when compared to normal digestion) and increased sensitivity (a lower pain threshold) have been widely considered to be the dominant factors in most cases of IBS. Probiotics can also influence both of these factors. Research shows that probiotics may reverse the hypersensitivity in the GI tract by protecting the tissues against harmful bacteria and other microorganisms, enhancing the strength of this barrier so that harmful bacteria and toxins cannot pass through to the bloodstream.[11] This direct effect on the tissue is in addition to the previously described effects on regulation of immune function that works to keep inflammation in check. Most recently, researchers have also found that some lactobacillus strains may stimulate cells in the tissues that respond to powerful pain relievers, to provide pain relief directly.[12] Research suggests that the subtle levels of gut inflammation can also affect brain functioning, at times leading to conditions such as depression.[13,14] These findings are exciting and need much further evaluation to really understand the multiple ways these bacteria may be helping to relieve the pain and cramping that come with IBS.

Since probiotics appear to have the ability to reverse unhealthy inflammatory responses, researchers are now studying whether probiotics can also reverse the results of these responses that can occur at sites in the body far removed from the GI tract. Some studies have shown decreases in inflammatory processes in the liver and even in the joints. This suggests that probiotics could be helpful for those who suffer from some of the non-GI conditions often associated with IBS, such as fibromyalgia and fatigue.

Probiotics As A Treatment for Other Conditions of the GI Tract

A number of scientific and clinical studies have also demonstrated that probiotics can reduce symptoms of various other conditions of the GI tract. What follows is an overview of some of those conditions.

Probiotics and Diarrhea

Rotavirus is a cause of infectious diarrhea in children. Globally, it claims more than 600,000 lives annually. Several studies have shown that some probiotic strains can be effective in reducing the duration of rotavirus-induced diarrhea, resulting in quicker recovery times and a potential decrease in deaths caused by the disease.

Diarrhea can also be caused by the use of antibiotics. A combined analysis (meta-analysis) of nine double-blind, placebo-controlled clinical trials indicated that certain probiotics (specifically *S. boulardii*, *L. acidophilus and bulgaricus*, *Enterococcus fecium SF68*, *Bifidobacterium longum*, and *Lactobacillus GG*) can help prevent this type of diarrhea. Certain bacterial strains in probiotics can also protect against diarrhea caused by *C. difficile*, a particularly pathogenic microorganism found in 20 percent of cases of antibiotic-associated diarrhea. One theory is that probiotic bacteria work by breaking down the chemical toxins produced by *C. difficile*. *S. boulardii*, a probiotic that is not a strain of bacteria but is instead a type of yeast, has shown protective activity. The bacterial probiotic strain *Lactobacillus GG* has been shown to prevent recurring episodes of *C. difficile*-associated diarrhea.[15] Other studies have even suggested that non-toxic strains of the *C. difficile* bacteria may prevent diarrhea associated with the toxic strain in 87 to 97 percent of patients.

Inflammatory Bowel Disease/Ulcerative Colitis/ Crohn's Disease

The rationale for the use of probiotics in IBD and its complications, such as pouchitis and post-operative recurrence of Crohn's disease, involves the disruption in the balance between "friendly" and harmful GI bacteria as well in how well the gut's immune system can differentiate "good" from "bad." There is a strong suggestion that IBD patients may be recognizing "good" bacteria as being "bad" and, as a result, develop what becomes a harmful inflammatory response.

Studies with a number of probiotic strains have shown a significant anti-inflammatory effect in experimental models of colitis. In a very small randomized trial, fewer (3 of 11) patients fed with bifidobacterium-fermented milk developed worsening of symptoms compared with 9 of 10 in the control group. In another small pilot study, 70.8 percent of 24 ulcerative colitis patients with mild to moderate clinical flare-up attained remission after treatment with *S. boulardii* for four weeks.

Research also indicates that the combination of an antibiotic with a high concentration of probiotics can decrease severe recurrence of Crohn's disease following surgery. For example, in one study that compared the combination of probiotics and the drug mesalazine with mesalazine alone, the rates of severe recurrence of Crohn's disease at one year were 20 percent among patients in the combination group compared to 40 percent in the mesalazine-only group.

Bacterial Overgrowth and Bacterial Migration Beyond the Lower Bowel

Studies of various probiotic preparations have shown that probiotics can also check the growth and spread of harmful bacteria to places in the GI tract where they do not normally reside. In one study of children with bacterial overgrowth associated with a medical condition called short bowel syndrome, the probiotic strain *Lactobacillus plantarum 299V* was found to prevent or delay the recurrence of digestive symptoms following antibiotic treatment. In a randomized, double-blind trial of 12 patients with chronic diarrhea related to bacterial overgrowth, the probiotic organisms *Lactobacillus casei* and *Lactobacillus acidophilus* helped reduce the diarrhea. The researchers recommended that these probiotics be administered on a continuous basis in this patient population. However, these studies were small and the results of other studies have not demonstrated the same benefits, so this is still controversial.

As the above studies show, probiotics can play an important role in preventing and treating various types of GI conditions. Now that we have explored this role, let's turn our attention to a new probiotic strain that is clinically proven to manage digestive upsets and to provide particular benefit for IBS. This probiotic strain is called Bifantis (*Bifidobacterium infantis* 35624, see photo below) and will be discussed in Chapter 5.

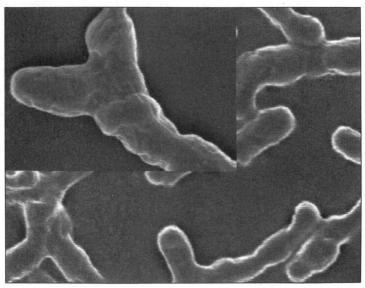

Bifidobacterium infantis 35624 (Bifantis)

Bifantis®:
A Unique Probiotic Strain

Recently, clinical trials have shown that the bacterial strain *Bifidobacterium infantis* 35624, or Bifantis®, can benefit people with IBS and other conditions of the GI tract. This chapter will discuss the clinical trials with this probiotic strain that have been published in *Gastroenterology* (March 2005) and *The American Journal of Gastroenterology* (July 2006), and provide some insights into how this probiotic can be combined with other strategies to manage digestive upsets including IBS.

Benefits of Bifantis in Irritable Bowel Syndrome

Two clinical efficacy trials were conducted on Bifantis for IBS. The first of these studies (considered a "pilot" study) compared the effects of two probiotic strains (Bifantis and *Lactobacillus salivarius*) on symptoms in patients with IBS.[7] In this study, 77 IBS patients (both men and women) received Bifantis, *L. salivarius*, or placebo for eight weeks. Patients taking Bifantis had significantly more relief than the lactobacillus and placebo groups from each of the main symptoms of IBS (abdominal pain/discomfort, distension/bloating, and difficult bowel movement), and the Bifantis group had better quality of life. Furthermore, Bifantis was well tolerated and did not cause any adverse side effects. At the same time, stool frequency or form changed little, so the improvements could not be attributed to either a laxative or an anti-diarrheal effect. Equally significant, in the patients treated with Bifantis, the ratio of IL-10/ IL-12 (anti-inflammatory/pro-inflammatory) cytokines increased, approaching that of the healthy volunteers, whereas there was no such change in the other treatment groups. The importance of these cytokines was discussed in Chapter 4.

The first study was followed by a larger, four week study of Bifantis in 362 female IBS patients between the ages of 18 and 65.[16] Again, all of the symptoms of IBS (abdominal pain/discomfort, bloating, sense of incomplete evacuation, straining, urgency, passage of gas and mucus, and bowel habit satisfaction) significantly improved in the Bifantis group. Furthermore, a global assessment of IBS symptoms (a question that asks "Have you had adequate relief of your IBS symptoms, yes or no?") at the end of therapy revealed a greater than 20 percent therapeutic benefit for Bifantis over placebo—the strongest therapeutic benefit in any IBS study, with any treatment, to date. Interestingly, patients taking Bifantis also had normalized bowel movement frequency, regardless of whether they started with very frequent (diarrhea) or very few (constipation) bowel movements. This appears to be a unique finding since other agents used or tested in IBS have tended to target only one type of IBS (diarrhea or constipation) but not work in both. Because these changes in bowel frequency were accompanied by significant improvement in the individual symptoms, such as pain and bloating, these findings indicate that the health benefits of Bifantis are not limited to any specific IBS subtype, but that it is effective for the entire spectrum of IBS patients. "We are pleased and excited with the results of this study, as it represents an advance in the treatment of IBS, which can cause such embarrassing symptoms, often on a daily basis," said Dr. Peter Whorwell, Professor of Medicine and Gastroenterology at the University of Manchester (UK) and lead author of the study.

> "We are pleased and excited with the results of this study, as it represents an advance in the treatment of IBS, which can cause such embarrassing symptoms, often on a daily basis,"
>
> —Dr. Peter Whorwell

While neither of these studies directly compared this probiotic with any other type of therapy, we can compare the individual trials and the therapeutic gain for each treatment reported in those studies to understand the relative benefits. The therapeutic gain is the percent

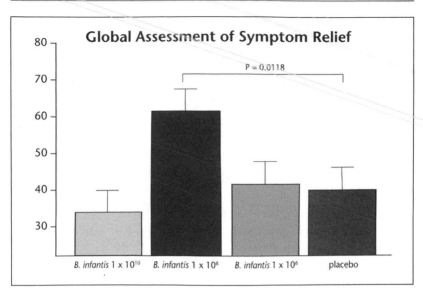

Comparison of effects of placebo and *Bifidobacterium infantis* 35624 on Subjects Global Assessment (SGA) of IBS symptoms. Positive response rates recorded at week 4, at the end of therapy. Subjects responded "yes" or "no" to the following question: *Please consider how you felt in the past week in regard to your IBS, in particular your general well-being and symptoms of abdominal discomfort or pain, bloating or distension, and altered bowel habit. Compared to the way you felt before beginning the medication, have you had adequate relief of your IBS symptoms?*[16]

increase that a treatment provides for a certain benefit (for example, pain relief) over the percentage provided by placebo. This therapeutic gain for Bifantis over placebo (20%–25%) for the global response score is comparable to—or greater than—those reported for the drugs Tegaserod and Alosetron (10%–20%). Therefore, this study with Bifantis provides clear evidence that it is beneficial for people with IBS.

The results of these two studies in IBS have been independently confirmed by a group of researchers at the University of Michigan in Ann Arbor. This review, which was presented at the American College of Gastroenterology conference in Philadelphia, Pennsylvania in October 2007, compiled data using a statistical technique called "meta-analysis." The analysis included 13 studies on the safety, effectiveness, and tolerability of probiotics for treating IBS. It found that only the Bifantis studies "used appropriate study design." The researchers commented that with the exception of the *Bifidobacterium infantis* 35624 studies, most studies were not designed in a way that made the data possible to validate, with limitations such as poor study design, inadequate blinding, inadequate trial length, inadequate sample size, and lack of proper analysis. Also, several studies failed to report results on tolerability and adverse events. The report stated ". . . the only probiotic to demonstrate significant improvement in IBS symptoms in appropriately designed studies was *Bifidobacterium infantis* 35624 [Bifantis]."

> *". . . the only probiotic to demonstrate significant improvement in IBS symptoms in appropriately designed studies was Bifidobacterium infantis 35624 [Bifantis]."*

Darren Brenner, MD, lead investigator on the meta-analysis project, added, "There is growing interest in medical and patient communities about the use of probiotics in IBS and lots of data has been published about this topic, but it's helpful to know the quality of that data before making a treatment decision. Our analysis showed that only this particular strain of probiotic, *Bifidobacterium infantis* 35624, has valid data for successfully treating IBS symptoms. At this point, we just don't have enough valid data to determine if other probiotics are effective for IBS."

Other Benefits of Bifantis

The benefits of Bifantis extend beyond IBS to other functional GI complaints. These complaints can happen all at once (like in IBS) or may be experienced individually. Bifantis is also beneficial for many common and recurring GI complaints, including:

- Abdominal pain
- Bloating
- Constipation
- Diarrhea
- Flatulence (gas)

When taken once a day on an ongoing basis, Bifantis can improve and maintain normal digestive function in people who suffer from such GI complaints, and help to prevent them from occurring in the first place in people who are already healthy.

Summary

Increasing evidence supports the critical role of the gut flora in a variety of functions that sustain our overall health. Central to this beneficial interaction between gut flora and the human body is the communication of the gut bacteria with the body's immune system and, in particular, with the immune components within the gut. Research has shown that when the gut flora or its interaction with the immune system becomes disturbed or imbalanced, disease can soon follow. Into this landscape comes a new player: the probiotic. Probiotics can benefit healthy people as well as those suffering from various diseases and conditions, most notably illnesses characterized by diarrhea, some inflammatory bowel diseases, and certain infectious disorders.

IBS can now be added to this list. Research into post-infectious varieties of IBS and the reporting of low-grade inflammation and immune activation in IBS patients indicate that imbalances in the GI flora can contribute to IBS. This evidence supports the use of probiotics for IBS, most particularly the probiotic strain *Bifidobacterium infantis* 35624, which is trademarked as Bifantis.

It is clear that the role of the gut flora is of great importance in IBS as well as in other GI illnesses. As clinical evidence of the effectiveness of probiotics for treating IBS and other GI conditions continues to emerge, a review of available trials emphasizes the importance of the right probiotic strain and the proper probiotic quantity. Equally important is the viability of the probiotic strain, meaning that the strain must survive passage through the stomach and small intestine so that it arrives alive in the colon. With regard to

IBS, the only probiotic strain that is clinically proven to meet these criteria is Bifantis. Although future research is needed to further define how probiotics can restore gut flora balance and manage IBS, existing scientific research suggests that Bifantis is a safe and effective treatment option for preventing and resolving IBS symptoms.

OTHER STEPS YOU CAN TAKE
TO HELP PREVENT DIGESTIVE UPSET

In addition to considering the use of Bifantis or other probiotic supplements, here are some other guidelines you can follow to improve and maintain your digestive health.

- Eat slowly, chewing your food thoroughly before swallowing.

- Avoid overeating or skipping meals, both of which can create digestive disturbances.

- Become aware of your personal "trigger foods" (foods that can cause discomfort) and avoid them, especially when traveling or dining out.

- Avoid eating foods that contain additives such as fructose and sorbitol.

- Minimize your intake of foods that are fried or high in fat.

- Include adequate amounts of fiber in your diet, according to what your system can tolerate.

- Drink plenty of water throughout the day, but restrict or eliminate your intake of alcoholic, caffeinated, and carbonated beverages.

- Avoid chewing gum, which can lead to the swallowing of air and abdominal distention.

Frequently Asked Questions

How do probiotics work?

Probiotics work by helping to re-establish the body's naturally occurring bacteria in the GI tract, also known as gut flora. This task is accomplished by probiotics' ability to reverse imbalances of the types of bacteria in the digestive system.

Are probiotics safe?

Yes. The safety of the bacteria used in the manufacture of probiotic supplements has been confirmed through more than 100 years of scientific research and experience.

Can I consume probiotics naturally from foods?

Yes. When cultured milk-based products are supplemented with probiotics, this ensures the growth of good bacteria in products such as yogurt, cottage cheese, and buttermilk. Fermented vegetables such as sauerkraut and soybeans (miso) are also natural probiotics. Unleavened sourdough breads also create a favorable environment for the development of healthy gut flora.

Do probiotics stimulate the immune system?

It appears so. Researchers are discovering that friendly bacteria not only promote digestive health but may also stimulate a healthy immune system by crowding out harmful bacteria as well as by generating "friendly" signals to our immune system.

Why should I take probiotics?

Probiotics offer a safe and effective way for you to restore the natural balance of your digestive system, especially if you suffer from constipation, diarrhea, abdominal discomfort, urgency, gas or bloating. Studies have demonstrated that probiotics can provide relief for some sufferers from inflammatory bowel disease (Crohn's and ulcerative colitis) and irritable bowel syndrome (IBS). Probiotics are also recommended for anyone taking an antibiotic drug in order to normalize and re-populate the gut flora destroyed by the antibiotic. Probiotics are also suggested for reducing the recurrence of vaginal yeast infections and for normalizing high cholesterol levels.

Are all probiotics the same?

No. Experts believe the benefits of probiotics depend on the type and dose of strain. They recommend that all probiotic strains be independently tested and evaluated in clinical trials. Although a variety of probiotic supplements have been shown to be useful for treating a variety of common digestive and GI problems, only *Bifidobacterium infantis* 35624, trademarked as Bifantis, is clinically proven to be effective for managing symptoms of IBS.

How do I differentiate probiotic strains?

Look for the specific name of the probiotic strain. There should be three parts to any bacterial name: the genus, species and strain. The strain designation is needed to track publications and history of use to verify that it is safe and has been shown to have probiotic benefits.[17]

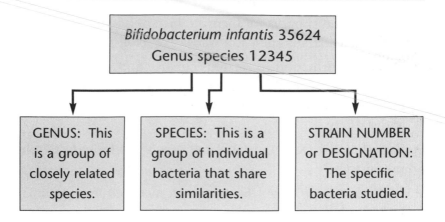

How do I choose a probiotic?

Clinical trials have shown that the strain and the quantity of bacteria are the key factors to consider when choosing a probiotic. Consumers are urged to look for clinically proven probiotics produced by reputable manufacturers. Trials of *Bifidobacterium infantis* 35624 (Bifantis®), found in the probiotic supplement Align® from Procter & Gamble, for example, have provided evidence of its ability to help restore the balance of healthy bacteria in the digestive system.

When shopping for a probiotic product, consumers should check that the label includes all of the following information:

- **Actual strain(s) name and the quantity of probiotic bacteria** for each strain listed. The number of probiotic bacteria needed to be effective is strain- and product-form specific; more is not necessarily better.

- **"Best used by" date and a batch or lot code.** The code printed on an individual container serves as a reference number for the plant to track production information.

- **Company information.** Look for products manufactured by well-trusted companies who have a history of good clinical evidence and support for their products. Also look for corporate contact details such as a website or a toll-free number.

- Dosing information, directions for use and storage. Many products have complicated dosing regimens or directions, and the suggested storage conditions vary based on probiotic form and stability.

- Expectations: Does the label tell you what to expect from product use?

- Facts: The Supplement Facts, which include the nutritional and supplement information.

What can I expect if I decide to use Bifantis?

People respond individually to dietary supplements, including Bifantis, and everybody follows a slightly different adjustment curve. No matter where you start, as your body begins to naturally adapt to daily supplementation with Bifantis, you should see improvements.

In the first few days after beginning to use Bifantis, some people may notice a temporary increase in gas and/or bloating. This is normal and is a sign that their bodies are adjusting to healthy bowel function. Generally, such effects will go away within a few more days of use as Bifantis restores and maintains proper digestive balance.

How can I obtain Bifantis?

Bifantis is found in the probiotic Align, which is sold by Procter and Gamble. Align can be purchased in several ways. You can order it online by visiting www.AlignGI.com or by calling (800) 208-0112. You can also ask your local pharmacist to order it for you.

Resources

These patient support and professional organizations can provide additional information on probiotics and digestive health.

American College of Gastroenterology (ACG)
Website: www.acg.gi.org

American Gastroenterological Association (AGA)
Website: www.gastro.org

American Pharmacists Association (APhA)
Website: www.aphanet.org

International Foundation for Functional Gastrointestinal Disorders (IFFGD)
Website: www.iffgd.org

Irritable Bowel Syndrome Self Help and Support Group
Website: www.ibsgroup.org

For additional information on Bifantis or the probiotic supplement Align please visit:
www.Bifantis.com
www.AlignGI.com

Glossary

Abdomen: The portion of the body between the chest and the pelvis.

Antibiotics: Microorganisms produce chemicals called antibiotics, which can inhibit the growth of or kill other microorganisms. Antibiotics are used to fight infections.

Antidepressant: An agent that elevates the mood of a depressed patient.

Antispasmodic: A drug that relieves the spasm (contraction) of a muscle.

Anus: The last portion of the digestive tract, through which fecal material is excreted.

Bacteriocins: Bacteriocins are small proteins synthesized by a given strain of bacteria and that are deadly to bacteria from other strains.

Bifantis: Bifantis is the trademarked name for the probiotic strain *Bifidobacterium infantis* 35624. Bifantis is a natural probiotic supplement that works within the digestive system to restore and maintain the intestinal balance of helpful versus harmful bacteria. In so doing, Bifantis maintains normal digestive health.

Bile: Bile is a yellow-green fluid that is made by the liver and stored in the gallbladder. It passes through the common bile duct into the duodenum where it helps in the digestion of fat. The principal components of bile are cholesterol, bile salts, and the pigment bilirubin.

Biopsy: The removal of a sample of tissue for purposes of diagnosis.

Bloat: Digestive disturbance marked by accumulation of gas in one or more stomach compartments, giving the sensation of an enlarged stomach.

Bowel: One of the divisions, or sections, of the intestine.

Colitis: Inflammation of the colon.

Colon: The part of the large intestine extending from the cecum (the first portion of the large intestine) to the rectum; sometimes used inaccurately as a synonym for the entire large intestine.

Colonoscopy: Colonoscopy is the endoscopic examination of the large colon and the distal part of the small bowel with a CCD camera or a fiber optic camera on a flexible tube passed through the anus. It may provide a visual diagnosis and grants the opportunity for biopsy or removal of suspected lesions.

Colony-forming units: A measure of how many bacteria are capable of dividing to form colonies. One viable bacterium can form a single bacterial colony.

Chronic: A chronic condition persists over a long period of time, as opposed to being acute.

Cytokines: Small proteins that mediate and regulate immunity, inflammation, and hematopoiesis (formation of red blood cells). They are part of the process of cell-cell signaling.

Crohn's disease: Crohn's disease is a chronic inflammatory disease that primarily involves the small and large intestine, but it can affect other parts of the digestive system as well. Crohn's is characterized by ulceration in the inner surface of the bowel.

Diarrhea: Abnormal frequency of fecal discharges; the stools contain more fluid than normal.

Duodenum: The first section of the small intestine: it starts at the pylorus (outlet of the stomach).

Dysbiosis: A breakdown in the balance between species of "protective" versus "harmful" intestinal bacteria.

Dyspepsia: Impaired digestion; usually used to describe stomach discomfort during meals.

Electrolytes: Salts that conduct electricity and are found in the body fluid, tissue, and blood. Examples are chloride, calcium, magnesium, sodium, and potassium. Sodium is concentrated in the extracellular fluid and potassium in the intracellular fluid. Proper balance is essential for muscle coordination, heart function, fluid absorption and excretion, nerve function, and concentration.

Epidemiology: Epidemiology is the study of populations in order to determine the frequency and distribution of disease and measure risks.

Epithelium: A tissue composed of layers of cells that line the cavities and surfaces of structures throughout the body. Among other parts of the body, epithelial cells line the inside of the GI tract. Functions of epithelial cells include secretion, absorption, protection, transcellular transport, sensation detection, and selective permeability.

Esophagus: A muscular tube that passes down from the throat to the stomach.

Fibromyalgia: Fibromyalgia is a chronic condition causing pain, stiffness, and tenderness of the muscles, tendons, and joints. Fibromyalgia is also characterized by restless sleep, awakening feeling tired, fatigue, anxiety, depression, and disturbances in bowel function.

Flora: The population of microbes inhabiting the outside or inside surfaces of people (or other animals).

Gastroenterologist: A physician who specializes in diseases of the gastrointestinal tract.

Gut: Part of the alimentary canal: the term especially refers to part of the intestine.

Inflammation: Inflammation is the body's reaction to infection, irritation or other injury. The key features are redness, warmth, swelling, and pain. The inflammatory response directs immune system components to the site of injury or infection.

Inflammatory: Pertaining to or characterized by inflammation.

Inflammatory bowel disorder: Chronic inflammatory diseases of the gastrointestinal tract. There are two major types: Crohn's disease and ulcerative colitis.

Irritable bowel syndrome: A chronic, continuous, or remittent gastrointestinal illness characterized by frequent unexplained symptoms that include abdominal pain, bloating, and bowel disturbance.

Lumen: Refers to the channel within a tube such as a blood vessel or to the cavity within a hollow organ such as the intestine.

Microflora: A small or strictly localized flora population.

Motility (gut): The movement by peristalsis along the small intestine.

Mucosa: A layer of moist tissue that lines and protects particular organs and body cavities throughout the body.

Organic disease: A disease in which there is a structural change in some organ or tissue in the body.

Over-the-counter drug: A drug that can be purchased legally without a doctor's prescription.

Pathogen: An agent that causes disease. The term pathogen most commonly is used to refer to infectious organisms, which include bacteria (such as staphylococcus), viruses (such as HIV), and fungi (such as yeast).

Pathogenicity: Ability to produce pathogenic changes (disease).

Peristalsis: The movement of the esophagus, stomach, and intestine. The action of peristalsis moves like an ocean wave through the muscle. The muscle of the organ produces a narrow area; this narrowing travels slowly down the length of the organ and thus pushes food and fluid through the digestive tract.

Pouchitis: The ileoanal pouch ("pull-through") and the continent ileostomy (Kock pouch) eliminate the need to wear an external ostomy appliance. In each case, the surgeon uses part of the patient's small intestine to create an internal pouch for the storage of stool. Sometimes the mucosa, or lining, of this internal pouch becomes inflamed. This is known as "pouchitis." Symptoms are similar to ulcerative colitis: diarrhea, crampy abdominal pain, increased frequency of stool, bleeding, fever, dehydration, and joint pain.

Probiotics: Live microorganisms, which when administered in adequate amounts, confer a health benefit on the host.

Rectum: The distal portion of the large intestine, from the sigmoid colon (last portion of the colon) to the anus.

Serotonin: A neurotransmitter produced in the brain known to influence the functioning of the cardiovascular, renal, immune, and gastrointestinal systems.

Sorbitol: A sugar substitute that can be found in fruit, and is also made synthetically. Its structure is a six-carbon alcohol.

Stomach: The organ responsible for preparing food for digestion: it is a sac-shaped digestive organ that is located in the upper abdomen, under the ribs. The upper part of the stomach connects to the esophagus, and the lower part leads into the small intestine. When food enters the stomach, muscles in the stomach wall create a rippling motion that mixes and mashes the food. At the same time, juices made by glands in the lining of the stomach help digest the food. After about 3 hours, the food becomes a liquid and moves into the small intestine, where digestion continues.

Stool: Feces; solid waste.

Traveler's diarrhea: Diarrhea that results from infections acquired while traveling to another country. In general, travelers at risk for diarrhea come from industrialized nations and travel to high-risk areas that are primarily within developing or less industrialized nations of the world. The disease usually is caused by eating food contaminated with bacteria or, less commonly, with parasites or viruses.

Ulcerative: Pertaining to or characterized by ulceration.

References

1. International Foundation for Functional Gastrointestinal Disorders. About Irritable Bowel Syndrome. Available at www.iffgd.org. Last updated November 22, 2007. Accessed November 28, 2007.

2. Cash B, Sullivan S, Barghout V. Total cost of IBS: employer and managed care perspective. *Am J Manag Care* 2005; 11:S7–S16.

3. Gastrointestinal and Liver Disease, vol 2, 7th edition, Chapter 91. 1794.

4. Thompson WG, Dotewall G, Drossman DA, et al. Irritable bowel syndrome: Guidelines for the diagnosis. *Gastroenterology Int* 1989; 2:92–95.

5. US Food and Drug Administration Center for Drug Evaluation and Research. FDA Public Health Advisory: tegaserod maleate (marketed as Zelnorm) March 30, 2007. Available at: www.fda.gov/cder/drug/advisory/tegaserod.htm Accessed January 10, 2008.

6. Neal KR, et al. Prevalence of gastrointestinal symptoms six months after bacterial gastroenteritis and the risk factors for development of the irritable bowel syndrome: postal survey of patients. *BMJ* 71997; 314: 779–782.

7. O'Mahony L, McCarthy J, Kelly P, et al. A Randomized, placebo-controlled, double-blind comparison of the probiotic bacteria lactobacillus and bifidobacterium in irritable bowel syndrome (IBS): symptom responses and relationship to cytokine profiles. *Gastroenterology* 2005; 128: 541–551.

8. Whorwell PJ, Altringer L, Morel J, et al. Efficacy of an encapsu-

lated probiotic Bifidobacterium infantis 35624 in women with irritable bowel syndrome. *Am J Gastroenterology* 2006; 101: 326–333.

9. Plinio. *Naturalis Historia,* 77AD.

10. Report of a joint FAO/WHO expert consultation on evaluation of health and nutritional properties of probiotics in food including powder milk with live lactic acid bacteria. C rdoba, Argentina, October 2001. Available at: www.who.int/foodsafety/publications/fs_management/en/probiotics.pdf Accessed January 10, 2008.

11. Isolauri E, S tas Y, Kankaanpa P, et al. Probiotics: effects on immunity. *Am J Clin Nutr.* 2001 Feb;73(2 Suppl):444S–450S.

12. Rousseaux C, Thuru X, Gelot A, et al. Lactobacillus acidophilus modulates intestinal pain and induces opioid and cannabinoid receptors. *Nat Med.* 2007;13(1):35-7. Epub 2006 Dec 10.

13. Logan AC, Katzman M. Major depressive disorder: probiotics may be an adjuvant therapy. *Med Hypotheses.* 2005;64(3):533–538.

14. Goehler LE, Lyte M, Gaykema RP. Infection-induced viscerosensory signals from the gut enhance anxiety: implications for psychoneuroimmunology. *Brain Behav Immun.* 2007;21(6):721–726. Epub 2007 Apr 10.

15. Pochapin M. The effect of probiotics on Clostridium difficile diarrhea. *Am J Gastroenterology* 2000;95(1 Suppl):S11–13.

16. Whorwell P, Altringer L, Morel J, Bond Y, Charbonneau D, O' Mahony L, Kiely B, Shanahan F, Quigley EMM. Efficacy of an encapsulated *Bifidobacterium infantis* 35624 in women with irritable bowel syndrome. *Am J Gastroenterology* 2006;101:1581–1590.

17. Reid, G. Potential uses of probiotics in clinical practice, *Clin Microbial Rev* 2003; 16(4): 658–672.

Index

About the Author

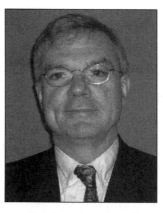

Eamonn M. Quigley, MD, FRCP, FACP, FACG, FRCPI, is a Professor of Medicine and Human Physiology at the National University of Ireland in Cork. He received his medical degree from the National University of Ireland and completed training in internal medicine and gastroenterology at the University of Glasgow; the Mayo Clinic; Hope Hospital, Salford; and the University of Manchester, United Kingdom.

Dr. Quigley's academic career began with a faculty appointment in the section of gastroenterology and hepatology at the University of Nebraska Medical Center, Omaha. He was an attending gastroenterologist at the University Hospital, the Veterans Administration Hospital, and Bishop Clarkson Memorial Hospital. After earning academic tenure and serving as chief of gastroenterology and hepatology at the University of Nebraska, he returned to Ireland in 1998.

His primary research interests and numerous publications have revolved around gastrointestinal motility, functional gastrointestinal disorders, and gastroesophageal reflux disease. Dr. Quigley served as editor-in-chief of the *American Journal of Gastroenterology* from 1997 to 2003 and is currently president of the World Organization of Gastroenterology (WGO-OMGE) and president-elect of the American College of Gastroenterology.